Diet Myths:
Sorting Through the Hype

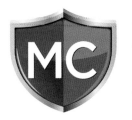

Mason Crest
450 Parkway Drive, Suite D
Broomall, PA 19008
www.masoncrest.com

Printed and bound in the United States of America.

First printing
9 8 7 6 5 4 3 2 1

Series ISBN: 978-1-4222-2874-6
Hardcover ISBN: 978-1-4222-2876-0
ebook ISBN: 978-1-4222-8938-9
Paperback ISBN: 978-1-4222-2991-0

The Library of Congress has cataloged the
        hardcopy format(s) as follows:

            Library of Congress Cataloging-in-Publication Data

Etingoff, Kim.
  Diet myths : sorting through the hype / Kim Etingoff.
    pages cm
  Audience: 10.
  Audience: Grade 4 to 6.
  ISBN 978-1-4222-2876-0 (hardcover) – ISBN 978-1-4222-2874-6 (series) – ISBN 978-1-4222-2991-0 (paperback) –ISBN 978-1-4222-8938-9 (ebook)
  1. Nutrition–Juvenile literature. 2. Diet–Juvenile literature. 3. Health–Juvenile literature. I. Title.
  RA784.E82 2014
  613.2–dc23
                        2013009445

Produced by Vestal Creative Services.
www.vestalcreative.com

UNDERSTANDING NUTRITION
A GATEWAY TO PHYSICAL & MENTAL HEALTH

Diet Myths:
Sorting Through the Hype

KIM ETINGOFF

Mason Crest

CONTENTS

INTRODUCTION
by Dr. Joshua Borus

There are many decisions to make about food. Almost everyone wants to "eat healthy"—but what does that really mean? What is the "right" amount of food and what is a "normal" portion size? Do I need sports drinks if I'm an athlete—or is water okay? Are all "organic" foods healthy? Getting reliable information about nutrition can be confusing. All sorts of restaurants and food makers spend billions of dollars trying to get you to buy their products, often by implying that a food is "good for you" or "healthy." Food packaging has unbiased, standardized nutrition labels, but if you don't know what to look for, they can be hard to understand. Magazine articles and the Internet seem to always have information about the latest fad diets or new "superfoods" but little information you can trust. Finally, everyone's parents, friends, and family have their own views on what is healthy. How are you supposed to make good decisions with all this information when you don't know how to interpret it?

The goal of this series is to arm you with information to help separate what is healthy from not healthy. The books in the series will help you think about things like proper portion size and how eating well can help you stay healthy, improve your mood, and manage your weight. These books will also help you take action. They will let you know some of the changes you can make to keep healthy and how to compare eating options.

Keep in mind a few broad rules:

- First, healthy eating is a lifelong process. Learning to try new foods, preparing foods in healthy ways, and focusing on the big picture are essential parts of that process. Almost no one can keep on a very restrictive diet for a long time or entirely cut out certain groups of foods, so it's best to figure out how to eat healthy in a way that's realistic for you by making a number of small changes.

- Second, a lot of healthy eating hasn't really changed much over the years and isn't that complicated once you know what to look for. The core of a healthy diet is still eating reasonable portions at regular meals. This should be mostly fruits and vegetables, reasonable amounts of proteins, and lots of whole grains, with few fried foods or extra fats. "Junk food" and sweets also have their place—they taste good and have a role in celebrations and other happy events—but they aren't meant to be a cornerstone of your diet!

- Third, avoid drinks with calories in them, beverages like sodas, iced tea, and most juices. Try to make your liquid intake all water and you'll be better off.

- Fourth, eating shouldn't be done mindlessly. Often people will munch while they watch TV or play games because it's something to do or because they're bored rather then because they are hungry. This can lead to lots of extra food intake, which usually isn't healthy. If you are eating, pay attention, so that you are enjoying what you eat and aware of your intake.

- Finally, eating is just one part of the equation. Exercise every day is the other part. Ideally, do an activity that makes you sweat and gets your heart beating fast for an hour a day—but even making small decisions like taking stairs instead of elevators or walking home from school instead of driving make a difference.

After you read this book, don't stop. Find out more about healthy eating. Choosemyplate.gov is a great Internet resource from the U.S. government that can be trusted to give good information; www.hsph.harvard.edu/nutritionsource is a webpage from the Harvard School of Public Health where scientists sort through all the data about food and nutrition and distill it into easy-to-understand messages. Your doctor or nurse can also help you learn more about making good decisions. You might also want to meet with a nutritionist to get more information about healthy living.

Food plays an important role in social events, informs our cultural heritage and traditions, and is an important part of our daily lives. It's not just how we fuel our bodies; it's also but how we nourish our spirit. Learn how to make good eating decisions and build healthy eating habits—and you'll have increased long-term health, both physically and psychologically.

So get started now!

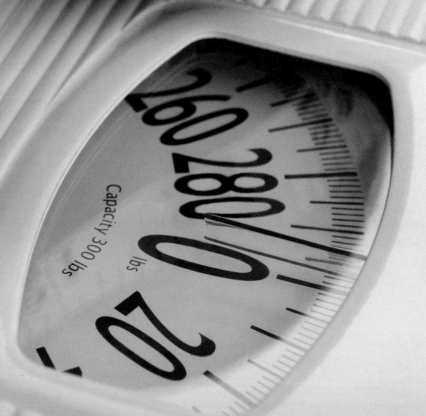

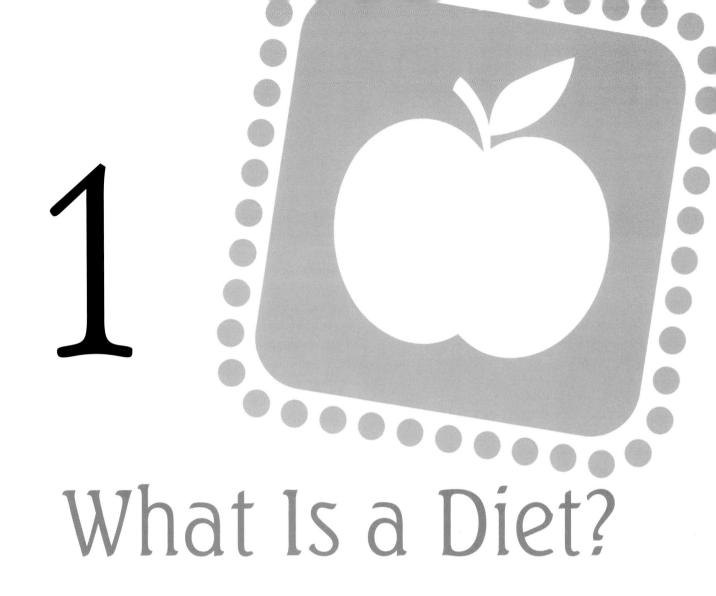

1

What Is a Diet?

Lots of people want to lose weight. Weighing too much is unhealthy. Too many pounds make us tired and sick, so a healthy weight is a good goal.

Some people turn to diets to lose weight. They follow a set of rules about how to eat. Diets can be very unhealthy though. Dieters have to be smart in order to make sure they're losing weight in a healthy way.

A Good Diet versus Dieting

The word diet means a couple of different things. Everyone has some sort of diet.

What's an Allergy?

When people are **allergic** to something, they have an allergy—which means that when they eat or touch or breathe a certain thing, their bodies react badly. They might sneeze or get a rash. They might get sick to their stomachs or not be able to breathe normally.

What's a Fad?

A **fad** is something—a style, for example, or a way of doing some-thing—that for a short time everyone is really excited about and lots of people do. Fads change all the time, and some of them can be pretty silly. In the 1600s in the Netherlands, tulips were so popular that people would pay 400 times what most people could earn in a year just to have a single tulip bulb! In the 1930s, swallowing live goldfish was a fad!

First of all, "diet" is just whatever you eat. Your diet is the foods you normally eat every day. Your diet could have lots of fruits and vegetables—or your diet might have a lot of meat in it. You might be **allergic** to nuts, and then your diet shouldn't have any nuts in it.

But "diet" can also mean a special way of eating to lose weight. The world is full of many different kinds of plans for losing weight. One kind of diet might tell you to eat more fruit, while another might tell you to stop eating bread. Another might only let you eat in the morning and afternoon, and not in the evening.

How can you tell which kind of diet people are talking about? Listen or read for clues. Sometimes people say they are "on a diet" or they say they "are dieting." That means the second kind of diet—eating to lose weight. If someone says, "What's your diet like?" they probably mean the first kind of diet, the way you normally eat.

Fad Diets

Fad diets are diets that are popular for just a short period of time. An author or scientist invents a diet they think will work or that people will follow. Then they write a book about it or they make a website about it. Other people hear about the new diet and think it's great. After a while, people often realize the diet doesn't work and isn't very healthy.

Usually fad diets are only popular for a few months or a couple of years.

People who go on fad diets want to lose weight. Losing weight can be hard because you have to eat healthy and you have to exercise. Diets seem like short cuts.

But fad diets don't work. You might lose weight, but then it all usually comes back when you stop dieting. Some people who go on fad diets don't lose any weight at all. Fad diets aren't healthy, since they don't give your body what it needs.

It's easy to spot fad diets. They promise you'll lose a lot of weight really fast. Most fad diets sound too good to be true. They usually are! They don't work.

The rules of fad diets sometimes tell you not to eat very much. If you stop eating enough food, you will lose weight, but there are good ways to lose weight and there are bad ways. Not eating enough is dangerous. All human beings need to eat food every day to be healthy.

Fad diets make you do **extreme** things. Some fad diets tell you certain foods are bad and tell you to stop eating them. One diet might tell you to stop eating all grains. Another will tell you to stop eating fruit. Both those diets are really bad ideas! The rules of a fad diet might also say one food is really, really good. They tell you to eat that food all the time, and maybe for every meal. Don't believe a diet when you have to eat one thing a lot, like grapefruit or boiled eggs with every meal.

What's the Point?

Diets are meant to help people lose weight. But why are people willing to do things like eat cabbage soup for every meal? People do some crazy things to lose weight.

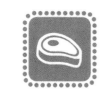

Extreme Diets

Here are some of the more unusual diets people have tried over the years. None of them are healthy.

- Grapefruit diet: People on this diet eat grapefruit at every meal. They believe that grapefruit helps the body burn fat.
- Cabbage soup diet: People on the cabbage soup diet eat cabbage soup for every meal. They aren't allowed to eat many other foods.
- Slimfast: Dieters are supposed to drink a Slimfast drink for breakfast and lunch every day. They can then have a small dinner.
- Atkins diet: You can eat as much meat, eggs, and cheese as you want, but you must cut out carbohydrates (bread, pasta, fruits, vegetables, and sugar).
- Breatharian diet: A very few people have tried to live only by breathing! They stop eating food. However, not eating is very dangerous, and people who follow this diet get sick and can even die.

If a person is overweight, he might want to lose weight really badly. He wants to look skinnier and fit into his favorite jeans. He mostly wants to feel good about himself.

A healthy weight is important, that's true. Many kids and adults do need to lose weight because they weigh too much. However, they need to lose weight in a healthy way that doesn't hurt their bodies. The whole point in losing weight is to be healthier. So it doesn't make sense to do that in a way that could hurt your health.

Diets often promise to help you lose weight really fast. Some say you'll lose ten pounds in a week! Or thirty pounds in a month! People who want to lose weight imagine what they'll look like in a week or a month on a diet. They're excited to think that they'll look and feel better so quickly. Diets seem like a quick fix.

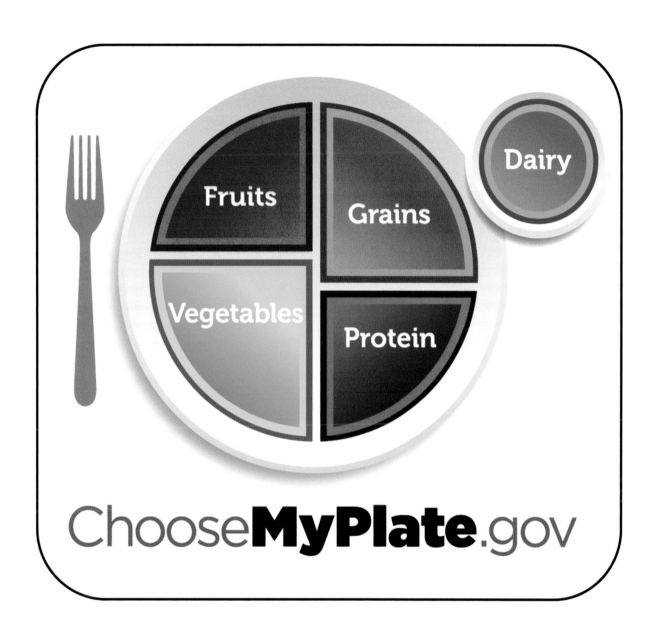

Diets that promise you can lose weight by only eating one thing aren't always healthy, and some are even dangerous. Governments around the world use different images to show their people how much of each kind of food they should be eating. The United States government uses MyPlate.

Think about it: if you had a choice between going on vacation in a week or waiting a year to go on vacation, which would you pick? Probably the vacation that's sooner, because you're so excited to travel. People diet for the same reason: because they don't want to wait. They want to lose weight as soon as possible.

It's definitely possible to lose weight in a healthy way. It takes longer though. You have to eat healthy foods. You have to exercise. It can take months or even years, depending on how much weight you need to lose. People get impatient and don't want to wait to lose pounds. Diets sound a lot better because they're faster.

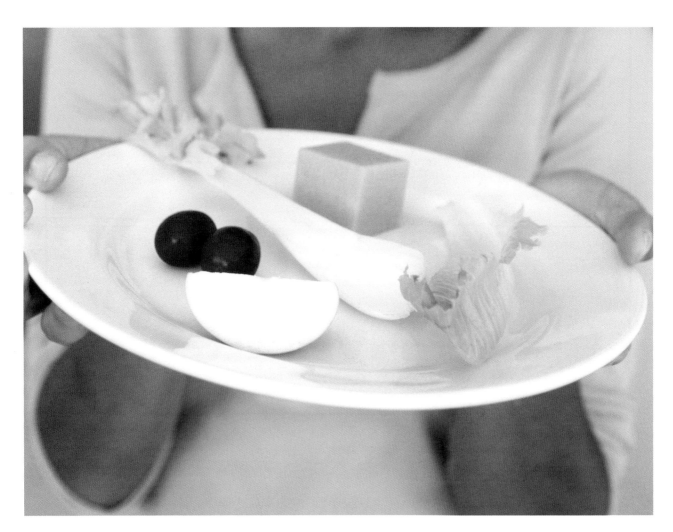

Eating too little and going on extreme diets aren't good for adults, and they're even worse for young people. There are healthier ways to get in shape than these extreme diets!

Vegetarians

People who don't eat meat are called vegetarians. For some people, not eating meat might seem like a weird or extreme way to eat. Vegetarianism is not the same as going on a diet though. Vegetarians don't cut out meat just to lose weight. They do it because they don't think eating animals is the right thing to do. Or because they feel better when they don't eat meat. Or because it's healthier for your heart. Vegetarianism is not a fad diet: it's healthy and people can eat vegetarian for years.

Young People and Diets

Young people almost never need to diet. They are growing and changing all the time. It's not normally a good idea to follow extreme rules about what you eat, especially while you're growing up. A lot of diets make you eat less food than is good for you.

Eating too little can be a bad idea for adults, and it's an even worse idea for young people. Dieting gets in the way of how you're growing and might mess with puberty later on.

Talk to your doctor if you think you need to lose weight. She'll help you decide if you really do need to lose weight, and then she'll help you figure out the best way to do it.

Getting smart about diets now is a good idea. You'll have to make lots of food decisions as you get older. What should you buy at the grocery store? Where should you go out to eat? How should you keep your weight at a healthy level? You'll have to answer all those questions and more.

The more you learn now about a good diet versus dieting, the better decisions you'll make as you grow older.

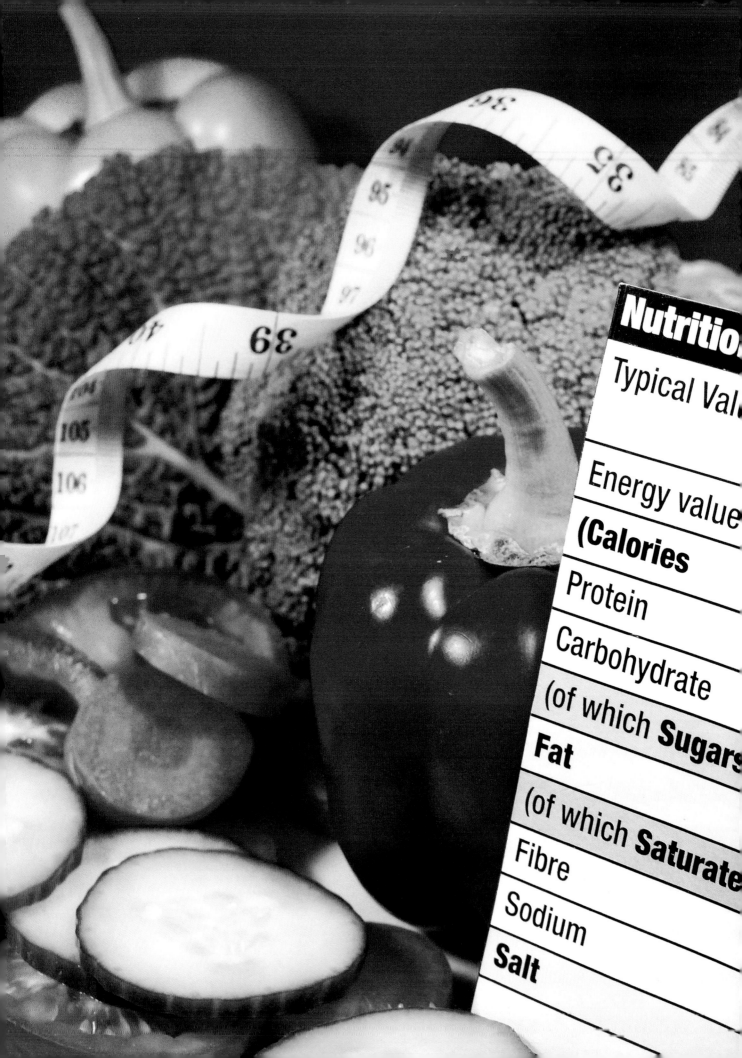

2

Popular Diet Myths

You can think of diets as rules. Diets are rules about what we can and cannot eat. They tell us when to eat, and when not to eat. They tell us how much we can eat. Diets often give us rules that are unhealthy or untrue. A lot of them are built on **myths**.

Myth #1:
"Carbohydrates Are Bad"

Carbohydrates are **nutrients** that give us energy. Different kinds of carbohydrates are in different foods. Sugar is one kind of carbohydrate, dietary fiber is another, and starches are a third kind.

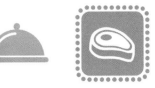

What's a Myth?

This word has a couple of different meanings. **Myths** are stories that explain the world for a group of people. For example, lots of cultures have myths that explain how the world was created. But myths can also be stories that lots of people believe that aren't true. Diet myths are stories about food and losing weight that lots of people think are true. However, once you look at the facts, you can see that the myths are false.

What Are Nutrients?

Nutrients are the things in foods that our bodies need to grow and stay alive.

What's Is Diabetes?

Diabetes is a disease caused by your body being unable to use sugar normally.

Some diets tell you that carbohydrates are bad and you shouldn't eat them. Dieters think their bodies just turn all carbohydrates into sugar, which gets turned into body weight.

What these diets don't tell you is that some kinds of carbohydrates are not as good as others. You shouldn't eat too much sugar, for example. Sugar leads to weight gain. Too much sugar can give you **diabetes** or make you sick in other ways.

Other kinds of carbohydrates are great for you! Vegetables and fruits have a lot of carbohydrates in the form of starch and fiber, and these things are good for you. Your body needs them. Whole grains have more good carbohydrates. You definitely shouldn't stop eating those foods.

Myth #2: "Fat Makes You Fat"

Other diets tell you to cut out fat. People often think eating fat makes you fat, so it make sense to stop eating fat.

Eating too much fat can lead to weight gain—but so can eating too much of anything else. You actually need some fat to live. Fat gives us energy and helps our bodies use vitamins.

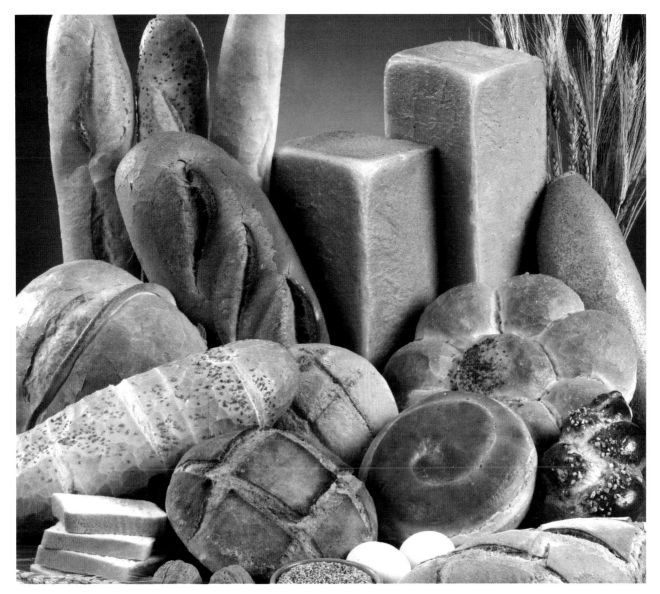

Carbohydrates can be found in many foods, including bread, pasta, and other foods made from grains. Some diets tell you not to eat any carbohydrates, but that's not a good idea.

Just like carbohydrates, though, there are good fats and not so good fats. Good fats are called unsaturated fat. Avocados, nuts, olive oil, and fish have unsaturated fat in them. Not-so-good fats are called saturated fats and trans fats. You should eat less of them because they can cause heart disease if you eat too much of them. Meat, butter, fried foods, and junk food have these unhealthy fats in them.

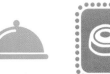

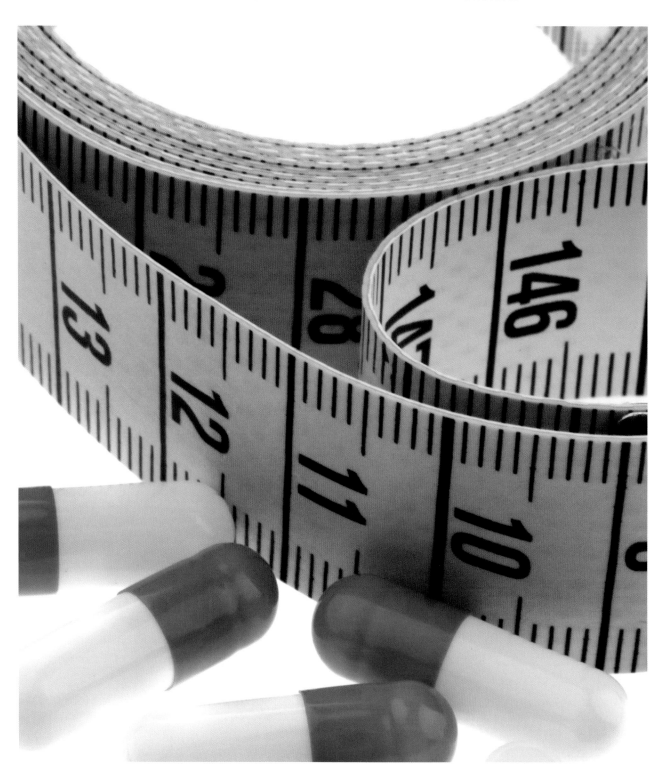

Taking pills that promise to help you lose weight is not a healthy way to get in shape or lose a few extra pounds. These pills don't help you lose weight and won't make you any more fit.

Myth #3: "'Natural' Means Healthy"

A lot of foods are labeled as "natural." Natural doesn't really mean anything, though, and it definitely doesn't mean a food is healthy. Any food company can use the word natural on its food, just to make people want to buy it.

Some food that is labeled as natural is unhealthy. You might find a box of pastries on the grocery store shelf that says it is natural. Does that mean you can eat as many pastries as you want? No! Even though they're "natural," they're still pastries with lots of sugar in them.

Don't worry too much about whether a food is natural or not. Pay attention to whether it has a lot of good nutrients (like vitamins and minerals). A lot of nutrients means it really is healthy!

Sometimes people try to lose weight with "natural" herbs. Taking a pill to lose weight sounds easy. If those pills are labeled as natural, they sound safe too.

You shouldn't try to lose weight with any kind of pill, though. Pills don't work. You should be eating healthy food instead. Besides, some natural pills can be dangerous. Stores used to sell an herb called ephedra, which promised to help people lose weight "naturally." Some dieters who took ephedra had heart attacks or died. Now the United States doesn't allow companies to sell ephedra.

Myth #4: "Skipping Meals Helps You Lose Weight"

Another diet myth is that you should lose weight by not eating so many meals. When you eat less food, you lose weight, which is true. But it's really unhealthy to skip entire meals.

If you really did skip lunch every day and ate the same amount as you normally did for breakfast and dinner, you would lose weight. (Don't do that though!) But that's not how it works for most people. Most people who skip a meal get really hungry. Later, they eat

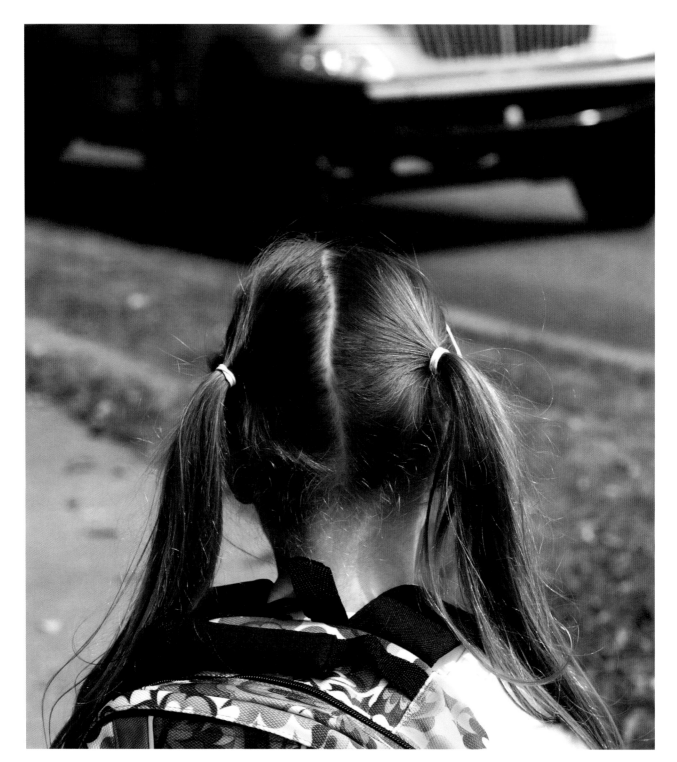

Heading to school without eating breakfast can leave you feeling tired, hungry, and sluggish all day. Eating a healthy breakfast before you leave in the morning is a good way to make sure you're ready for the day.

a lot more than they normally would have. They actually end up eating more food. They might even gain weight because they're eating so much to make up for skipping a meal.

Say you skip breakfast. You'll probably get really hungry before lunch. Imagine for lunch you normally eat a sandwich, some pretzels, a piece of fruit, and some milk. You skipped breakfast though, so you want to eat more because you're so hungry. You end up eating your normal lunch plus more. You might buy a bag of chips from the vending machine. Your friend gives you his graham crackers. And you buy an ice cream bar. All together, that's more food than you would have eaten at breakfast. You should have just eaten breakfast and lunch like usual.

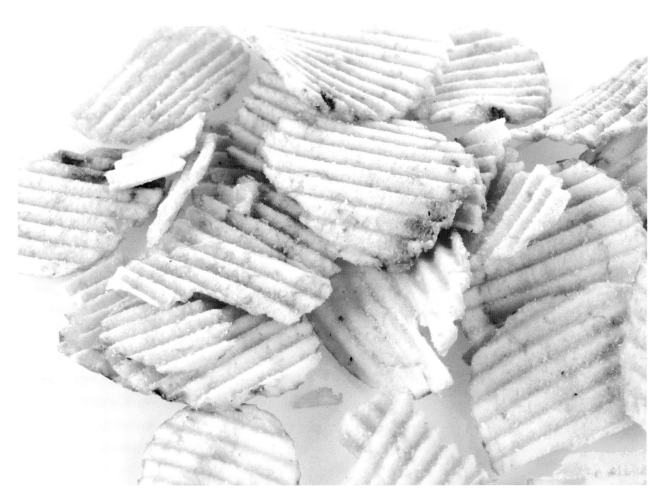

When you don't eat breakfast in the morning, you're more likely to choose sweet or salty snacks like chips later in the day.

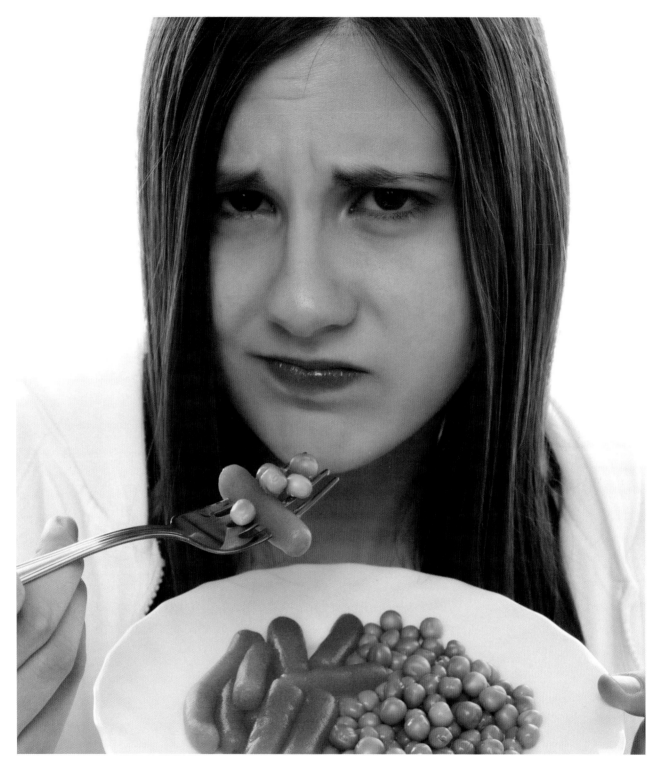

You won't always like every kind of healthy food, but finding healthy foods you like will make it easier for you to stay in shape and help you stick with making good food choices.

Myth #5:
"Healthy Food Tastes Bad"

Lots of young people think healthy food tastes bad. So losing weight or just being healthy means eating gross food.

Healthy foods can definitely be tasty! You just have to learn to like them. You have to try new foods. Healthy food usually tastes really good. Think about how good fresh fruits taste.

Not liking foods is okay. We all have different tastes. You have to give new foods a fair chance, though. If you think you don't like something but you've never actually tasted it, try it. You'll probably like it if you keep an open mind.

Keep an eye out for recipe books for healthy foods. Get your family to help you make some of the recipes that look the best. You'll be surprised at how good healthy food really is!

Spotting Diet Myths

You hear a lot about what to eat and what not to eat. You read about diet tips in magazines and online. You hear about diets on TV. Your school nurse, doctor, and parents give you health advice. How are you supposed to know if what you're hearing is a fact or a diet myth?

If it sounds too good to be true, it probably is a myth. Any diet that says you can lose weight in a very short time is a myth. You might read about scientific studies that talk about something that helps people lose weight. Although it's science, that study isn't the whole story. You should read more about other studies on the same thing. Then you'll get the whole picture. Finally, you can probably trust your nurse or doctor. They are trained in medicine, and can give you real information about losing weight.

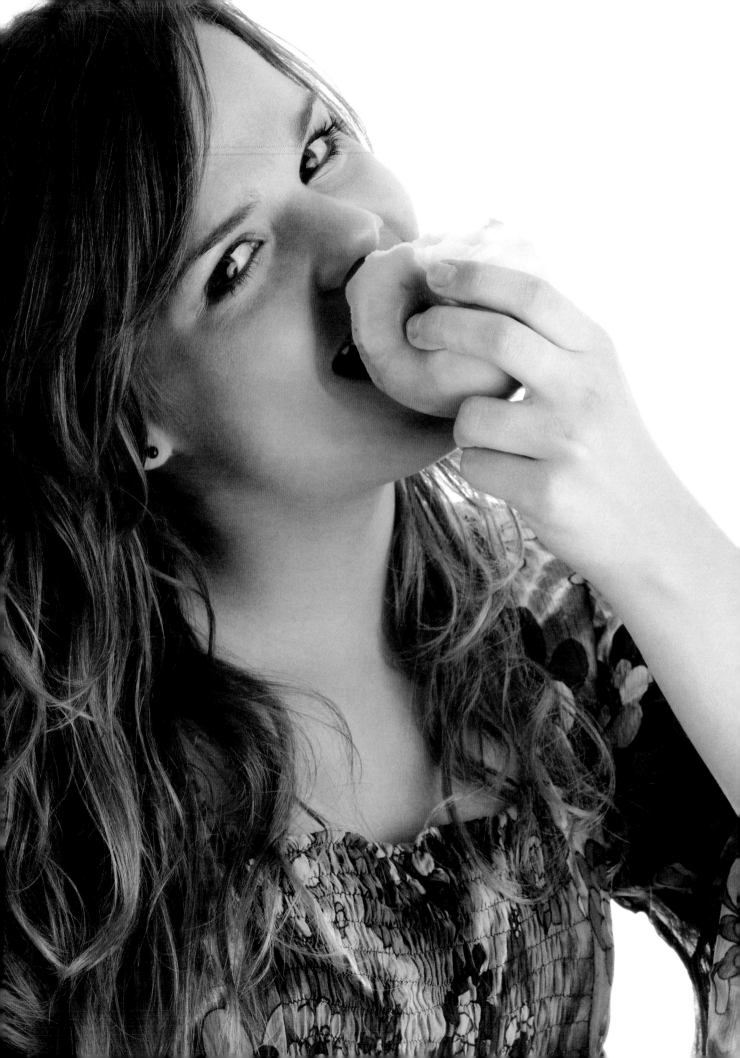

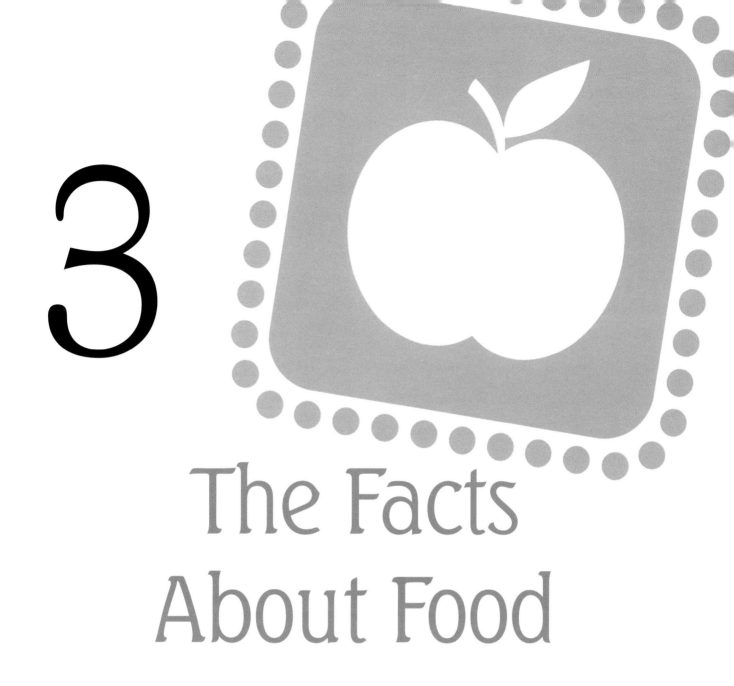

3

The Facts
About Food

Most diets out there aren't healthy. The only way to really lose weight and be healthy is to eat right and get exercise. Shortcuts just don't exist.

Why aren't diets healthy? For lots of reasons. The rules of diets don't allow people to eat enough food. They don't let you eat enough kinds of food. And they don't teach you the right things about food.

Breakfast

LOW-FAT YOGURT AND FRUIT — 250 CALORIES
CHOCOLATE DOUGHNUT — 270 CALORIES
WHOLE-GRAIN CEREAL WITH SKIM MILK — 140 CALORIES
BAGEL AND CREAM CHEESE — 450 CALORIES
* BISCUIT WITH SAUSAGE, EGG AND CHEESE — 570 CALORIES

Lunch

TUNA SALAD SANDWICH ON WHOLE WHEAT BREAD — 215 CALORIES
GRILLED CHICKEN WRAP — 250 CALORIES
GRILLED SALMON SALAD — 300 CALORIES
PIZZA (2 SLICES) — 540 CALORIES
* BURGER, FRIES, SODA (SMALL MEAL) — 839 CALORIES

Dinner

SALAD WITH TUNA — 300 CALORIES
GRILLED CHICKEN BREAST, BROWN RICE, AND VEGETABLES — 450 CALORIES
SPAGHETTI WITH TOMATO SAUCE — 450 CALORIES
7OZ SIRLOIN STEAK, STEAMED POTATOES, AND VEGETABLES — 550 CALORIES
* PIZZA (2 SLICES) — 540 CALORIES

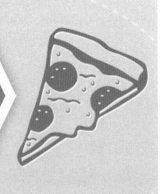

Keeping track of the calories you eat each day is a good way to make sure you're not eating more than you need.

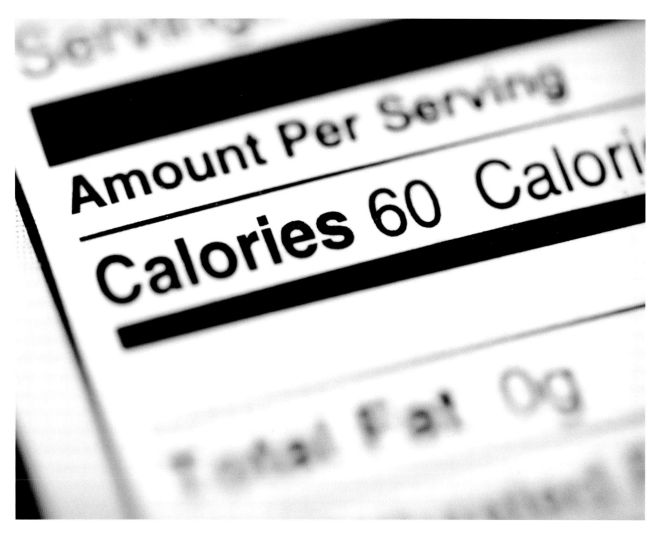

Check food labels to see how many calories are in one serving of the food you're eating.

Calories

All food gives us energy. We need to eat food to have energy to run around, go to school, and have a good time with friends. We need energy from food just to breathe, pump blood, and think. Without food, we couldn't do any of those things.

The energy in food is measured in calories. A hamburger with 500 calories has a lot of energy. An apple with 50 calories has a little bit of energy.

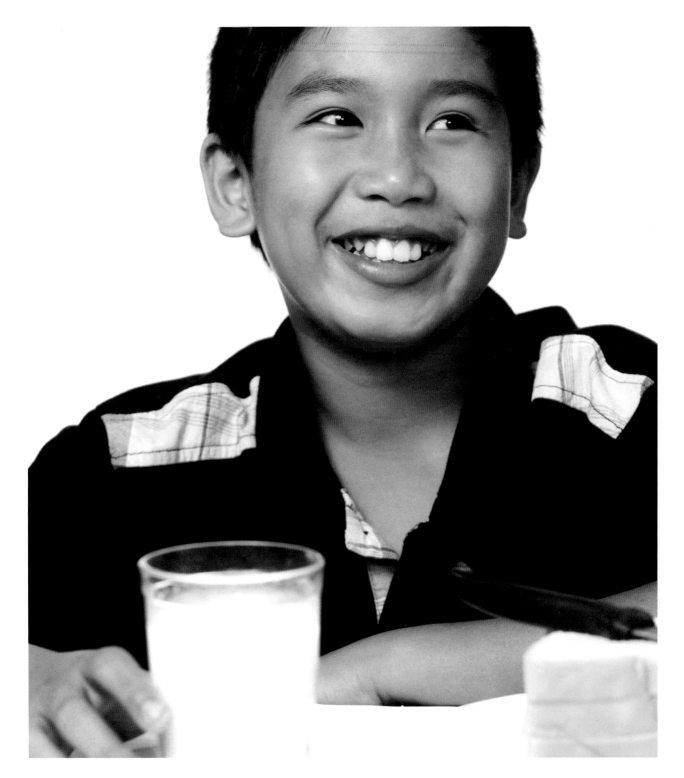

Milk and meat are good sources of protein. Some vegetarians have trouble getting enough protein if they don't eat meat or other animal foods.

A calorie is a measurement just like any other. Think about an orange. You could measure how wide it is in inches. You could weigh it on a scale in pounds. And you can measure its energy in calories.

Everyone needs about 2,000 calories every day. Some people need fewer calories, and some need more, but 2,000 is a good average. Bigger people usually need more calories. Boys normally need more calories than girls.

Calories have a lot to do with how much we weigh. When you eat more than 2,000 calories a day, you start to gain weight. When you eat less than 2,000 calories a day, you start to lose weight.

Diets work because eating fewer calories leads to weight loss. The safe way to lose weight is to eat a little fewer calories every day. There are safe ways to do that.

However, many diets tell us to eat a lot fewer calories every day. Instead of 2,000 calories, a dieter might only eat 1,500 or even less! Cutting out so many calories means cutting out a lot of food.

Remember, people need food to live. When we eat less food (and a lot fewer calories), we can get sick. We feel tired all the time. We don't have enough energy to learn or work or play sports or hang out with friends.

Many diets are unhealthy because they don't let you eat enough calories. Diets can make people hungry and tired. That's not a healthy way to lose weight! Besides, people don't usually stick with diets that make them feel bad. When that happens, people get discouraged and give up. They often end up gaining back all the weight they lost. They might even gain more weight back than they lost, so they end up weighing more than they did to start with.

Nutrients

All people need nutrients to live healthy lives. Nutrients are substances our bodies don't make on their own. We have to eat foods that have nutrients in them.

Nutrients do all sorts of things for our bodies. They help us grow up, give us energy, and keep your bones and muscles and skin healthy. Without enough nutrients, people get sick.

Nutrition Facts

Serving Size 1 container (226g)

Amount Per Serving

Calories 110   Calories from Fat 0

	% Daily Value*
Total Fat 0g	0 %
Saturated Fat 0g	0 %
Trans Fat 0g	
Cholesterol Less than 5mg	1 %
Sodium 160mg	7 %
Total Carbohydrate 15g	5 %
Dietary Fiber 0g	0 %
Sugars 10g	
Protein 13g	

Vitamin A	0 %	Vitamin C	4 %
Calcium	45 %	Iron	0 %

*Percent Daily Values are based on a 2,000 calorie diet. Your Daily Values may be higher or lower depending on your calorie needs.

Check food labels to see the amount of fat, sugar, protein, vitamins, and minerals in your food. Try avoiding high-sugar, high-fat foods.

The problem with special diets is that they don't give people enough nutrients. Many diets limit the kind of food you eat, and that limits the amount of nutrients you get.

Diets that don't let you eat enough protein get in the way of growing healthy muscles. You might not get enough protein if you stop eating meat and dairy products.

Diets that don't let you eat carbohydrates might keep you from getting enough nutrients too. When you don't eat any foods with carbohydrates, you miss out on eating the **vitamins**, iron, and other **minerals** that are also in those foods. For example, low-carb diets tell you not to eat potatoes, but potatoes are vegetables with lots of good things for you, and they are part of healthy eating.

You should be eating all sorts of healthy foods!

Your Attitude

Diets don't teach you the right way to think about food. You should feel good about food and eating. Food is tasty and it's a necessary part of life.

When people go on a diet, they start to think food is an enemy. Food means gaining weight to them. Or food means lots of hard-to-follow rules.

A better way to think about food is that it makes us healthy and strong. Those are good things to be. The kinds of foods that make us stronger and healthier are the foods we want to eat. Rather than forcing yourself to go on a diet, it's much better to think positively about food and come up with a healthy eating plan.

Vitamins and Minerals

People usually say "vitamins and minerals" in the same sentence, but they're two different things. Plants and animals make **vitamins**. For example, plants make vitamin A, and animals' bodies just naturally make vitamin B. **Minerals**, on the other hand, come from dirt and water. Plants and animals can't make minerals. But plants do suck them up from the dirt and water, and animals eat those plants. Then we eat the plants and animals, so we get the minerals too. Vitamins and minerals also have something in common: people's bodies can't make enough of them and we have to get both vitamins and minerals from food.

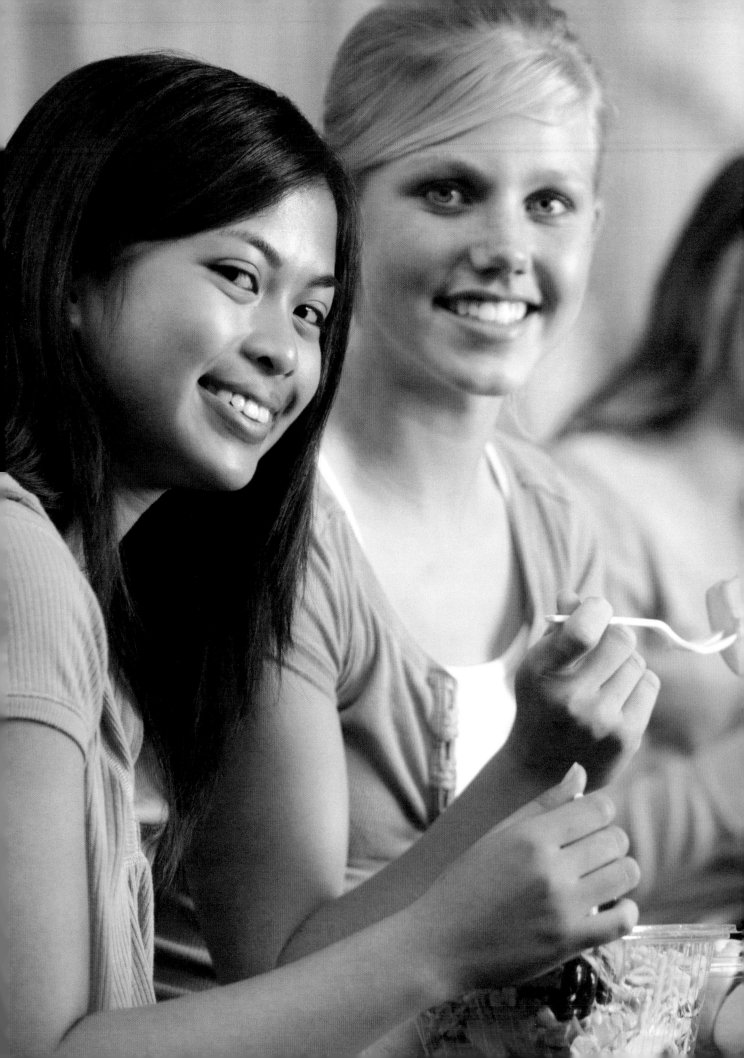

4

Diet Decisions

Diets aren't usually the healthiest way to eat. They don't really help you lose weight, and they don't keep you strong, **energetic**, and growing.

Diets don't teach you ways to eat that last a lifetime. Most people who diet end up gaining back any weight they lost. Diets are just too hard! Imagine having to eat a grapefruit with every meal for the rest of your life! Or never eating a piece of cake or a cookie again!

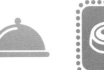

Healthy eating **habits** are much better than diets. Habits last your whole life. You only diet for a few weeks or months and then go back to how you ate before. Learning healthy habits now will keep you healthy for a long time! There are plenty of ways to control your weight and stay healthy without dieting.

Do You Need to Lose Weight?

The reason diets are so popular is because so many people think they need to lose weight. Not everyone needs to lose weight, though.

What Does "Energetic" Mean?

Someone who is **energetic** has lots of energy. They can run around and get things done without feeling tired.

What's a Stroke?

A **stroke** is when brain cells die because the blood flow inside the brain is interrupted so that the cells don't get the oxygen they need. A person who has had a stroke may not be able to speak or move normally. It depends what part of the brain was damaged by the stroke and how much of the brain was hurt. Very large strokes can kill people.

Plenty of people do weigh too much. When someone weighs a little too much, they are overweight. When someone weighs a lot too much, they are called obese. About one-fifth of the people in the entire world are overweight or obese. In other words, around the world, one out of five people weigh too much. In areas of the world like Europe and most of North America, one out of two people are overweight or obese. That means half of all the people who live in those areas need to lose weight.

Weighing the right amount is a great goal to have. You'll be healthier and happier and feel good about yourself. Weighing too many pounds leads to sickness, like heart disease, diabetes, and **strokes**. People who weigh too much have a hard time moving around, and they might not feel very good about how they look.

People feel a lot of pressure to weigh less. Sometimes people want to lose weight

What's a Habit?

A **habit** is something you've done so many times that you keep doing it without having to think about it. For example, brushing your teeth every night before you go to bed might be a habit. You don't have to think about it—you just do it. Or a not-so-good habit might be chewing your fingernails when you feel nervous. It's something else you do without thinking.

Good habits can help you out a lot in life. They help you do things that are healthy for you every day, without giving it a thought. They make it easier to do healthy things.

We usually have to make an effort to make new habits—but once we've made a new habit, then we can stop thinking about it. Some scientists say that we need to do something for at least a couple of months before it will become a habit. That means you'll have to think about making a change in your life every day for at least two months. It won't be easy. But once you have a new habit, it will help you for the rest of your life!

for health reasons, but sometimes the reason they want to be thinner is about wanting to look different. We usually only see skinny people on TV and in the movies. We think skinny is beautiful—but skinny doesn't mean healthy. Weighing too little is unhealthy too. Some people want to lose weight so they can be skinnier. However, they may already be a healthy weight. They don't need to lose weight to be any healthier. In fact, they might become less healthy when they lose weight.

How do you know if you're the right weight or not? Young people often find it especially hard to know if they're the right weight. They are still growing and their bodies are changing a lot.

Your doctor can help you figure out if you're the right weight. Doctors use a special number called a BMI (Body Mass Index) to tell if your weight is right. BMI is based on

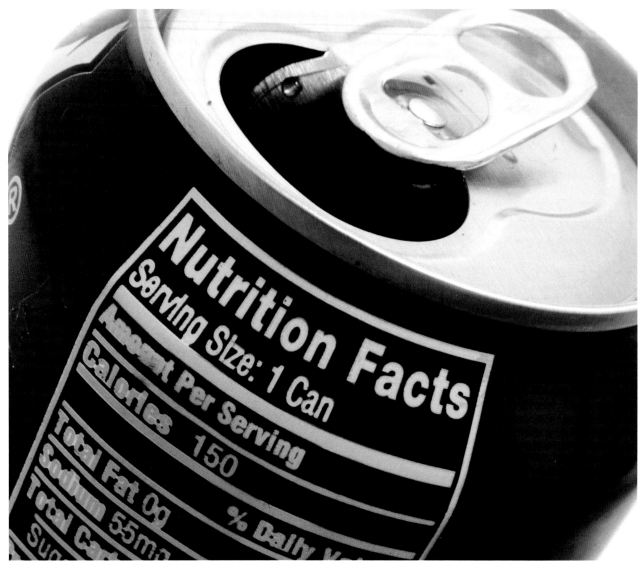

Soda is high in calories. Soda and other sugary drinks aren't very healthy and can lead to weight gain and health problems.

how tall you are and how much you weigh. If your BMI is too low, you don't weigh enough. If it's too high, you weigh too much. Right in the middle is a range of BMI numbers that are healthy.

If you're worried about your weight, go to your doctor. He'll be able to calculate your BMI. Then he can help you figure out what your BMI means and what to do if it's not in the healthy range.

Eating Disorders

People who take really extreme steps to be thin may have an eating disorder. Anorexia is one kind of eating disorder. People with anorexia stop eating and starve themselves on purpose to lose weight. Bulimia is another kind of eating disorder. People with bulimia eat but then make themselves throw up or exercise a lot to get rid of the calories they ate. Eating disorders are very unhealthy. People with eating disorders need to get help right away.

Losing Weight the Healthy Way

If your doctor says you would be healthier if you lost weight, you have some choices. You could go on a diet, and have to follow a lot of strict rules. You might be hungry all the time, and you might not get enough of the nutrients you need. Or you could learn healthier ways to lose weight.

Healthy weight loss programs will take longer. You will lose weight slowly. You'll also feel better because you will be eating all the things your body needs.

In order to lose weight, you have to cut down on calories. Diets make you cut them down by a lot every day. You really only need to cut them down by a little every day. Here are some ideas for doing that:

- Cut out at least one soda a day. The more sugary drinks you cut out, the better.
- Make your dessert smaller. Instead of a huge piece of cake, have a very small one. Or skip it altogether.

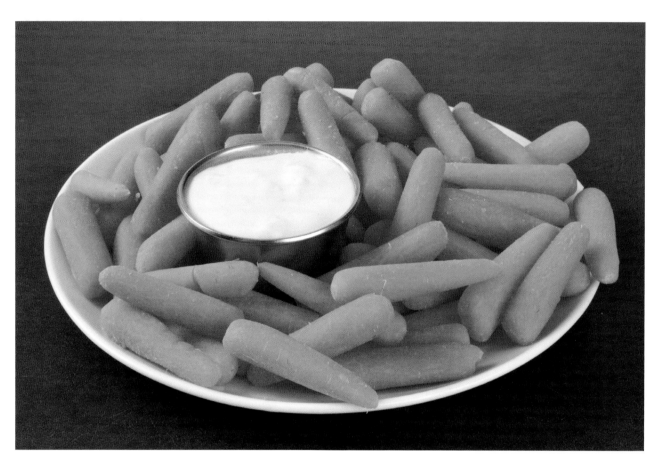

Switching a bag of chips or cookies for some carrot sticks is a good way to stay healthy while snacking between meals. Snacking isn't bad if you can eat healthier snacks.

- Give yourself small servings at dinner. If you finish everything on your plate, and you're still hungry, you can have more. If you're full, don't take more.
- Eat slowly so you give your body time to feel full. When you eat fast, you eat more food than your body really needs.
- Save junk food for special occasions. Don't eat chips, cookies, sugary cereal, and other junk foods every day. Replace them with fruits and vegetables.

When you're trying to lose weight, you can still eat in between meals. Healthy snacks are fine. If you're hungry between meals, you should eat a small snack. Make sure it's healthy and don't reach for ice cream or chips. A healthy snack might be carrot sticks or fruit. When you eat snacks during the day, you won't overeat at meals.

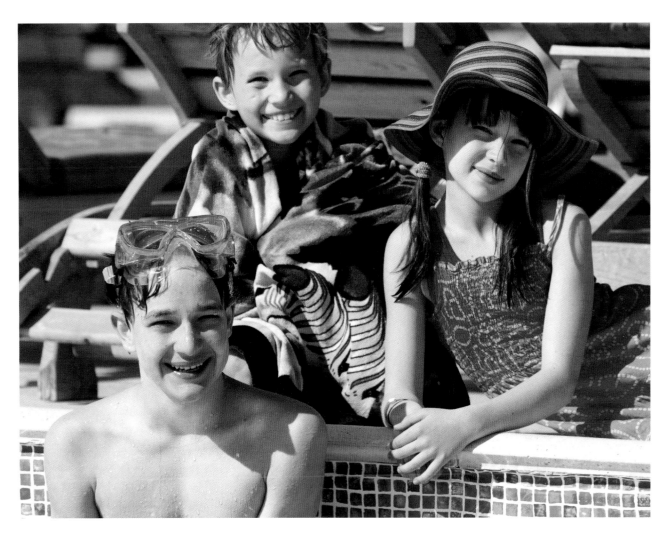

Playing sports, swimming, or even just walking outside can all be great ways to get active. Find something you have fun doing and you'll enjoy the time you spend exercising.

Of course, you have to exercise to lose weight in a healthy way. Exercise uses calories up, and it makes your heart, muscles, and lungs stronger.

Choose an exercise you like. Try running, swimming, hiking, or join a sports team. Then exercise a few times a week for at least a half-hour. More is better, but don't push yourself too hard. You don't want to get injured and have to sit on the couch for weeks!

You'll start to notice weight loss after you eat less calories and start exercising. Be patient, and pay attention to how you're feeling. Besides losing weight, you'll start feeling better and moving better.

Staying Healthy

Because young people's bodies are growing, they need a certain amount of calories. The best thing for them to do is to start eating healthy. They don't usually need to count calories or cut down on food. Eating the best, healthiest foods is the key to looking and feeling good.

EAT FRUITS AND VEGETABLES

You can never eat too much fruits and vegetables! Every meal you eat should have some fruits and vegetables in it.

For breakfast, eat some fruit with your cereal. For lunch, have carrot sticks, and salad, or tomatoes on your sandwich. For a snack, eat celery sticks and hummus or peanut butter. For dinner, make sure you take a big helping of vegetables.

Fruits and vegetables have lots of good nutrients in them. For example, citrus fruits like oranges have vitamin C. Vitamin C helps protect us from getting sick and helps heal wounds.

What Does "Refined" Mean?

Something that is **refined** has had something unwanted—like dirt or something else that people don't like—removed from it. People used to think that refined grains were better. They thought that white flour and white rice looked better and tasted better. In reality, though, refined grains have had the good stuff removed from them.

EAT WHOLE GRAINS

Grains are the seeds of some kinds of grass plants. Rice, wheat, oats, and barley are all grains. Grains are sometimes made into other foods. Wheat is ground up into flour, and flour is made into bread, crackers, and more. Oats are crushed up and made into oatmeal.

You can buy two different kinds of grains. Most of the grains we eat are called **refined** grains. Every grain seed that grows has three parts. Refined grains only have one of those three parts. They're missing two other parts, which have lots of good nutrients in them.

Whole grains have all three parts. Each seed is whole—that's why they're called whole grains. They have all the nutrients they possibly can.

You should try to eat as many whole-grain foods as possible. Whole-grain foods are usually darker than refined grain foods. Whole-wheat bread is made out of whole grains and is usually brown. White bread is refined and is lighter. Brown rice is a whole grain, and white rice is refined.

Even if you think you don't like whole grains, give them a try! You might find out that you do really like them. And they're part of a good diet.

Mix It Up

Diets are unhealthy because they limit how many kinds of foods you eat. To be healthy, you should eat as many kinds of food as you can! Don't just eat one thing. Mix it up!

Food is divided up into food groups. Our bodies need some foods from each of those groups every day: fruits, vegetables, grains, protein foods (meat, eggs, beans, tofu), and dairy. A healthy diet has all of those food groups. Each food group is good for you in a different way. When we eat them all together, we get as much good stuff as we can from all the groups.

You should eat food from all the groups every day. Think about what you eat now. Do you eat from every group? If not, try to fit in what you're missing.

Stay Away from Junk Food

A good general rule is to limit how much junk food you eat. Junk foods are foods that don't have many good nutrients. They usually have too much sugar and salt. Too much sugar and salt is unhealthy and can make you sick over time.

We're used to eating junk foods. You can find them in the grocery store, at school, and in your cupboard at home. You eat them with friends, for lunch at school, and as an evening snack.

Junk food is okay once in a while. We eat it because it tastes good! You won't be very happy if you never get to eat it. And no food is so bad that you can't ever eat it. The trick is to not eat it as much. Let yourself have those foods once in a while—but not every day.

Not eating junk food doesn't mean you have to go hungry. Just replace some of the junk foods you normally eat (or drink) with healthier foods. Choose water or 100 percent fruit juice instead of soda. Eat carrots and dip instead of chips.

A SIP OF SODA: HOW SOFT DRINKS IMPACT YOUR HEALTH

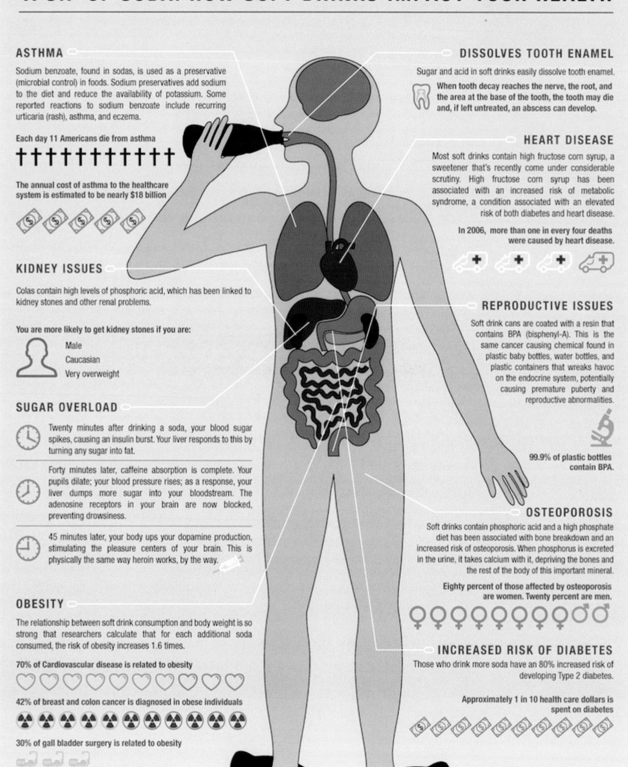

ASTHMA

Sodium benzoate, found in sodas, is used as a preservative (microbial control) in foods. Sodium preservatives add sodium to the diet and reduce the availability of potassium. Some reported reactions to sodium benzoate include recurring urticaria (rash), asthma, and eczema.

Each day 11 Americans die from asthma

The annual cost of asthma to the healthcare system is estimated to be nearly $18 billion

KIDNEY ISSUES

Colas contain high levels of phosphoric acid, which has been linked to kidney stones and other renal problems.

You are more likely to get kidney stones if you are:

Male
Caucasian
Very overweight

SUGAR OVERLOAD

Twenty minutes after drinking a soda, your blood sugar spikes, causing an insulin burst. Your liver responds to this by turning any sugar into fat.

Forty minutes later, caffeine absorption is complete. Your pupils dilate; your blood pressure rises; as a response, your liver dumps more sugar into your bloodstream. The adenosine receptors in your brain are now blocked, preventing drowsiness.

45 minutes later, your body ups your dopamine production, stimulating the pleasure centers of your brain. This is physically the same way heroin works, by the way.

OBESITY

The relationship between soft drink consumption and body weight is so strong that researchers calculate that for each additional soda consumed, the risk of obesity increases 1.6 times.

70% of Cardiovascular disease is related to obesity

42% of breast and colon cancer is diagnosed in obese individuals

30% of gall bladder surgery is related to obesity

DISSOLVES TOOTH ENAMEL

Sugar and acid in soft drinks easily dissolve tooth enamel. When tooth decay reaches the nerve, the root, and the area at the base of the tooth, the tooth may die and, if left untreated, an abscess can develop.

HEART DISEASE

Most soft drinks contain high fructose corn syrup, a sweetener that's recently come under considerable scrutiny. High fructose corn syrup has been associated with an increased risk of metabolic syndrome, a condition associated with an elevated risk of both diabetes and heart disease.

In 2006, more than one in every four deaths were caused by heart disease.

REPRODUCTIVE ISSUES

Soft drink cans are coated with a resin that contains BPA (bisphenyl-A). This is the same cancer causing chemical found in plastic baby bottles, water bottles, and plastic containers that wreaks havoc on the endocrine system, potentially causing premature puberty and reproductive abnormalities.

99.9% of plastic bottles contain BPA.

OSTEOPOROSIS

Soft drinks contain phosphoric acid and a high phosphate diet has been associated with bone breakdown and an increased risk of osteoporosis. When phosphorus is excreted in the urine, it takes calcium with it, depriving the bones and the rest of the body of this important mineral.

Eighty percent of those affected by osteoporosis are women. Twenty percent are men.

INCREASED RISK OF DIABETES

Those who drink more soda have an 80% increased risk of developing Type 2 diabetes.

Approximately 1 in 10 health care dollars is spent on diabetes

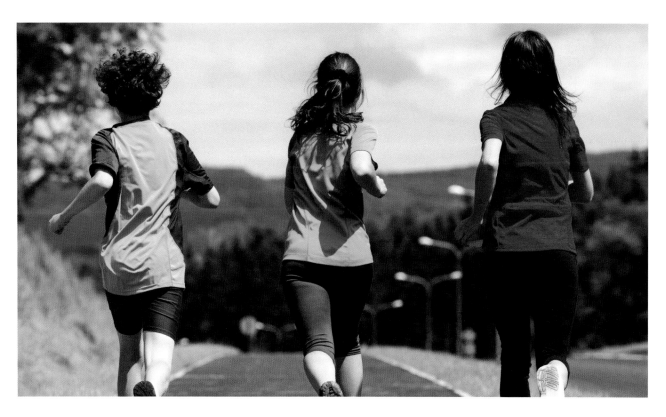

Eating right and getting plenty of exercise is the best way to stay healthy and watch your weight. If you need to lose weight, exercise and healthy food are the only real path to fitness.

EXERCISE

Staying healthy is all about eating healthy, but don't forget about exercise. Moving around is really good for you, and it's something that most of us don't do enough.

As a young person, you have lots of chances to exercise. Take swimming lessons. Play on a soccer team. Take walks with your friends or family. Dance. Ride your bicycle.

Whatever you do, move! Anything is better than sitting in front of the TV or computer for hours every day. You can still do those things, but get some exercise too.

Create your own healthy eating plan! The only secrets to weight loss are to eat healthy foods, don't eat too much, and exercise. You don't need diets to tell you exactly what and how to eat. Just use your common sense—and you'll be on your way to living a happy and healthy life.

Find Out More

ONLINE

Calorie Count
caloriecount.about.com

Healthy Eating Games
pbskids.org/games/healthyeating.html

KidsHealth: Is Dieting OK for Kids?
kidshealth.org/kid/stay_healthy/food/diet.html

MyPlate
www.choosemyplate.gov

IN BOOKS

Kajander, Kathleen. *Be Fit, Be Strong, Be You.* Minneapolis, Minn.: Free Spirit Publishing, 2010.

Katzen, Mollie. *Honest Pretzels and 64 Other Amazing Recipes for Kids Who Love to Cook.* Berkeley, Calif.: Tricycle Press, 2009.

Pollan, Michael. *The Omnivore's Dilemma; The Secrets Behind What You Eat, Young Readers Edition.* New York: Dial Books, 2009.

Index

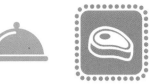

About the Author & Consultant

Kim Etingoff lives in Boston, Massachusetts, spending part of her time working on farms. Kim has written a number of books for young people on topics including health, history, nutrition, and business.

Dr. Borus graduated from the Harvard Medical School and the Harvard School of Public Health. He completed a residency in Pediatrics and then served as Chief Resident at Floating Hospital for Children at Tufts Medical Center before completing a fellowship in Adolescent Medicine at Boston Children's Hospital. He is currently an attending physician in the Division of Adolescent and Young Adult Medicine at Boston Children's Hospital and an Instructor of Pediatrics at Harvard Medical School.

Picture Credits